The TRINITY Detox: 21 Days To Becoming HealthyWealthy

DR. LAJOYCE BROOKSHIRE

Naturopath, Doctor of Naturopathic Ministry,
Master Herbalist, Licensed & Ordained Pastor

Renewing Your Mind Ink
A Division of Renewing Your Mind Foundation, Inc.
315 Dartmouth Drive, Unit 535
Marshalls Creek, Pennsylvania 18335

Cover Designed by: ENIGMA GRAPHICS
Cover Photography by: Lady Abstract
Interior Layout by: TWA Solutions.com

ISBN: 978-1-58441-009-6

Library of Congress Control Number: 2025918558

For Humanity

This book is dedicated to all who are
sick and tired of being
Sick AND Tired

In Memory Of

Joana Mae Wallace Hunter-Baker
John Morris Hunter
Marilyn Enyard-Hunter
Claudette Dyches
Rev. Patricia "Patsy" Moore Brigham
Betty Wallace
Constance Montgomery
Larry Esposito
Ruthie Newell

Also by *Dr. LaJoyce Brookshire*

*Ask The Good Doctor: Kitchen Warriors 101 -
Homemade Healthy*

*Ask The Good Doctor: The Detox Edition Remixed For A
Healthy New You*

*Ask The Good Doctor: Happy New Year, Healthy New
You (The Detox Edition)*

*Ask The Good Doctor: Yes, You Are What You Eat -
Recipes To Enhance Your Wellness Journey*

*Women Behind The Mic: Curators of Pop Culture
Volume One "Word To The Wise"*

*Women Behind The Mic: Curators of The Culture
Volume Two "The Hip-Hop Edition"*

The Last Listening Party of The Notorious B.I.G.

Faith Under Fire: Betrayed By A Thing Called Love

Web of Deception
Soul Food

Contributor:
Detox Or Die

GhettOver Girls

Souls of My Sisters

*Souls Revealed: A Souls of My Sisters Book of Revelations and
Tools for Healing Your Life, Soul, and Spirit*

ACKNOWLEDGMENTS

I give all honor, glory, and praise to God, from whom all blessings flow. I am thankful for having been blessed with a thirst for knowledge about health. I did not even know it was something for which I was thirsty until my friend Cyndi Rodgers gave a persuasive speech about health when I was a senior in high school. Something in my spirit resonated deeply with me that day, and the fire has continued to burn hotter and hotter, causing an insatiable quest to learn all I can and share it with the world.

It is a dream come true to be able to present TRINITY as a solid solution to a problem that has plagued mankind. I want to thank the following people who have made contributions to my being able to continue this work:

My exceptional husband, Gus—Your level of understanding of my need to crisscross the globe to teach about better health practices is not just admirable, it is love, and I know it. Who loves you, Bay-bee?

My daughter, Brooke—Thank you for being my Angel Baby and a shining example of the HealthyWealthy Life. You have been pouring chlorophyll for friends and family since you were a tot! I cannot wait to experience your next chapter. Love you!

To my best friend in the whole wide world, my best friends, and prayer warriors—You keep me fortified, aligned, and accountable. Y'all know who you are!

My team—Irvin Wright-IW (Supervising Producer): Thank you for your solid guidance, your "Let's Get It" posture, and rocking and rolling with me for the last, I-don't-know-how-many years. Thomasina Perkins (PR), Cheryl Hines (Voice Overs), Jessica Tilles (Editor), Harry Lawson (Enigma Graphic Design), and Ken Johnson (Mean Ol Lion Media Podcast Production)—your talents are deeply appreciated and help me hold all things together.

To T-Que Winning—Your ability to share what and whom you have access to is so beautiful. I am here with TRINITY because of your unselfishness. From sharing a phone number to jumping on a plane to meet me halfway around the world to share an idea, you are PROOF that women can work together well when they lead with love and respect. Thank you, Little Sister!

To my EDMARK Family—Thank you for welcoming me into the fold, catching the TRINITY vision, and respecting the naturopathic mantle. Chairman Sam, you are appreciated for integrating me into a well-established system and being a great business mentor.

To the Wellness Warriors, past, present, and future—As long as God gives me breath, I will continue in this work for you all.

In His Service…Dr. LaJoyce

TABLE OF CONTENTS

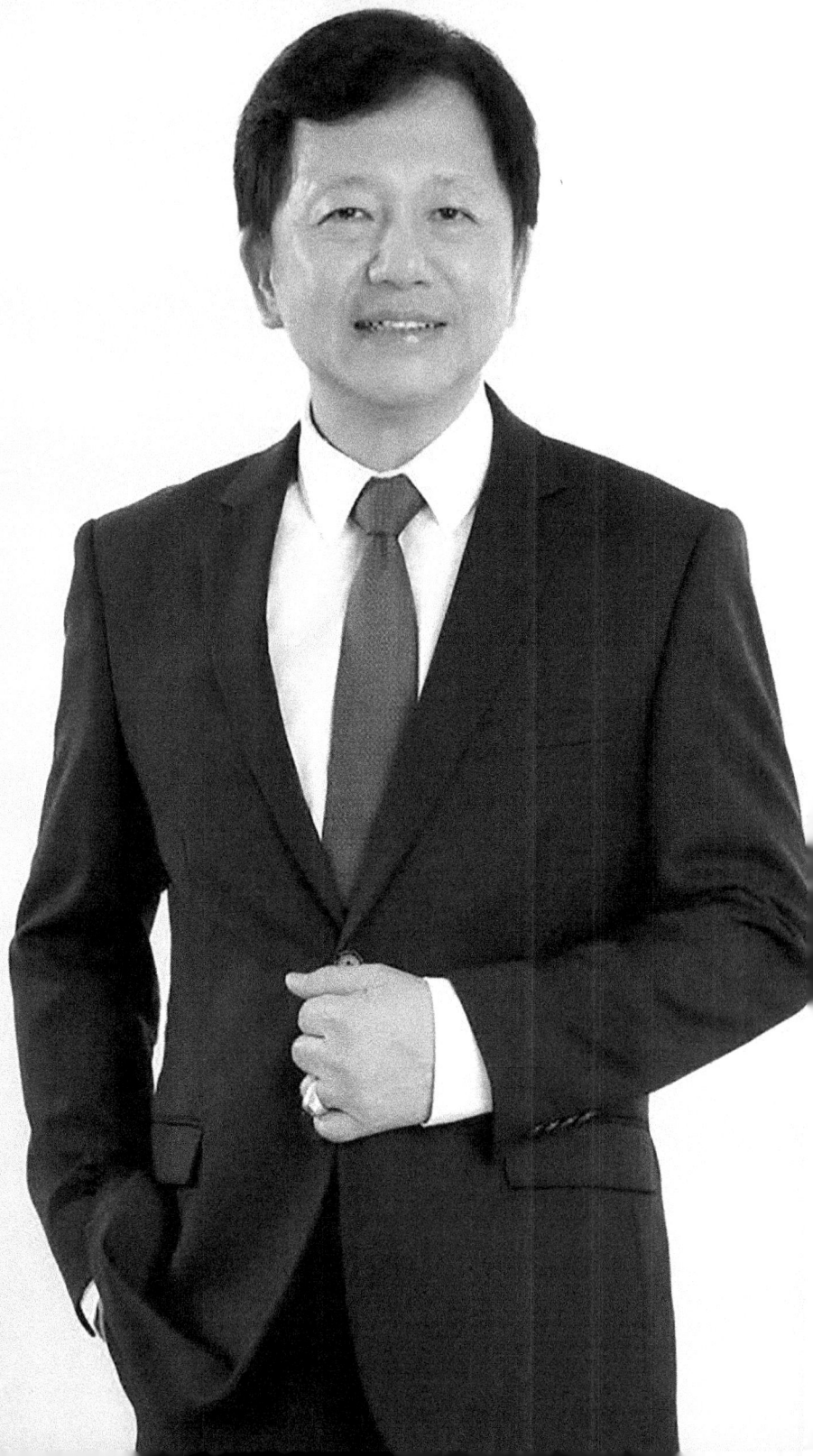

FOREWORD

When TRINITY was presented to us by Dr. LaJoyce Brookshire, it was more than just a product idea—it was a calling. In a world where health is often sacrificed for convenience and wealth is pursued at the expense of well-being, we envisioned a solution that could harmonize both. TRINITY was born from this vision: to restore balance, vitality, and hope to those seeking a better way of living.

I will never forget the moment I crossed paths with Dr. LaJoyce Brookshire. Her deep understanding of natural health, her integrity, and her relentless pursuit of truth immediately resonated with me. What began as a conversation quickly evolved into a powerful collaboration—one rooted in shared values, mutual respect, and a deep desire to serve humanity.

Dr. LaJoyce brought something extraordinary with the TRINITY mission: a voice of clarity in a noisy world and a healer's heart that beats for transformation. This book, *The TRINITY Detox: 21 Days to Becoming HealthyWealthy*, is a natural extension of her life's work. It combines scientific insight with spiritual wisdom, and personal testimony with practical guidance. On these pages, you will find answers. More importantly, you will find empowerment.

As the founder of EDMARK, I have seen firsthand how TRINITY is changing lives. From cellular health to emotional well-being, from detoxification to rejuvenation, the testimonies are undeniable. This book captures that impact and equips every person to experience it for themselves. It is my deepest honor to support this important work.

I believe this book will not only educate and inspire but also ignite a movement toward total wellness—body, mind, and soul.

To Dr. LaJoyce, thank you for your brilliance, your faith, and your unwavering commitment to excellence. Together, we have not just launched a product—we are lighting the way for a healthier, wealthier world. Let the transformation begin.

"When purpose meets partnership, miracles happen."

Sam Low
Founder & Chairman
EDMARK Group International

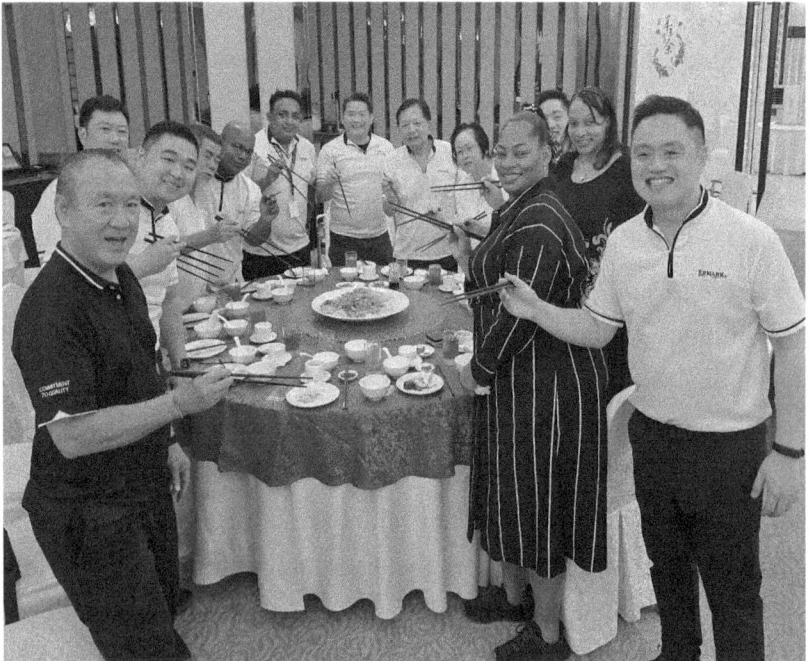

Being Welcomed into The EDMARK family with an unforgettable meal in Malaysia.

INTRODUCTION

A Personal Invitation to Healing

*"Let us cleanse ourselves from every
defilement of body and spirit..."*
–2 Corinthians 7:1

It was April of 2020, at the height of global quarantine, when I found myself crying daily as the world was assaulted by an invisible enemy named COVID. I watched in horror as the ticker rose, counting the lives lost in my city and across the globe. I was devastated to see this giant disease toss humanity around like a rag doll.

I took to the SiriusXM airwaves with my show *Ask The Good Doctor*, sharing the vital, life-saving information I held in my hands. It was information I knew could help the people who needed it most. I was determined not to allow this "Goliath" of a virus to destroy us. I showed up on countless Zooms, television and radio programs, church platforms, corporate wellness meetings, and family gatherings.

In a world where wellness is overpriced, overcomplicated, and gatekept, I wanted to give people something radical. That is when the lightbulb came on to make available a high-quality product line to help everyone that I had personally been utilizing for years. The company I chose initially was not equipped to handle the shipping.

My frustration turned hopeful when God whispered to me… Not yet. It was a promise that delays are not denials.

I was ready to jump in to help in every way possible, but as the entire globe sat at a screeching halt, I remembered a powerful truth we lived by when I worked in the entertainment industry: "Stay ready, so you don't have to get ready." I know now, without question, that because I had clung to this posture of readiness—not just in business but with my health—the life I saved was my own.

Here is my true story:

In January 1992, I was living the dream life in New York City, thriving in my dream career in the entertainment industry, and I was happy and full of energy. My skin was radiant, I slept soundly, and my digestion was clockwork. Headaches? None. Aches and pains? Not a single one. By all accounts, I had never felt healthier.

Then suddenly, everything changed. The stress of an intense life event collided with the daily rigors of fast-paced New York living, and my body began to scream for help. I was unwell, and it was not just a passing cold or fatigue. My digestion came to a screeching halt. My skin was breaking out. And I was waking at all hours of the night. My issues were not just deep—they were systemic. My medical doctor and alternative therapy doctor, Frederick Douglas Burton, saw it before I did and gently, then persistently, encouraged me to complete a detox program.

"Who, me?" I scoffed.

"Yes, you," he insisted.

Even though I was Miss Herbs and Miss Pro-Organic-Everything, I resisted—until a nasty bronchial infection seemingly came out of nowhere (after years of study, I now know exactly how the bronchitis took hold). I tried everything in my natural medicine cabinet, but after weeks of suffering, I succumbed to purchasing two rounds of antibiotics at $80 a pop. Still, the infection lingered. And suddenly, I realized that although I looked healthy on the outside, I was a toxic mess on the inside.

Kicking and screaming, I surrendered to the detox. And within 48 hours, something remarkable happened: my clogged ears popped open. My cough quieted. My breathing was easier. Then came the purge—thick, multi-colored mucus from every orifice. Foul breath. Funky armpits. Eye crust. Earwax. And yes, the infamous green-tinged toilet visits. Gross? Absolutely. But also, glorious.

By Day 21, I felt like brand new money. My energy surged. My skin glowed. My sleep deepened. My sugar and salt cravings vanished. My bowel movements were regular, odorless, and healthy. And perhaps most miraculous of all, I felt lighter emotionally. The burdens I had carried from that recent life trauma shifted. I had clarity. I had hope. I had peace.

That first detox was not just a physical cleanse…it was a rebirth.

I now perform this spiritual and physical renewal at the beginning of every season. As a Naturopathic Doctor, I have guided countless others through this same path, watching them recover from disease, doubt, and dysfunction as they too reclaimed their wellness.

This book is your invitation:

To attain. To maintain. To reclaim. To become HealthyWealthy with the TRINITY 21-Day Detoxification Program co-created by EDMARK International and myself. It was obedience that I listened when God whispered Not yet during the quarantine, because I am blessed to be in partnership with the greatest company ever. What seemingly looked like a delay led me to destiny. The discovery led me halfway around the world to Malaysia and a partnership that will last for generations.

I say to you… no more sitting on the sidelines of wellness. No more being "wellness adjacent." It is time to take the plunge, because the secret to living the healthy life you crave begins with one word: **Detox**.

Welcome to the TRINITY Experience!

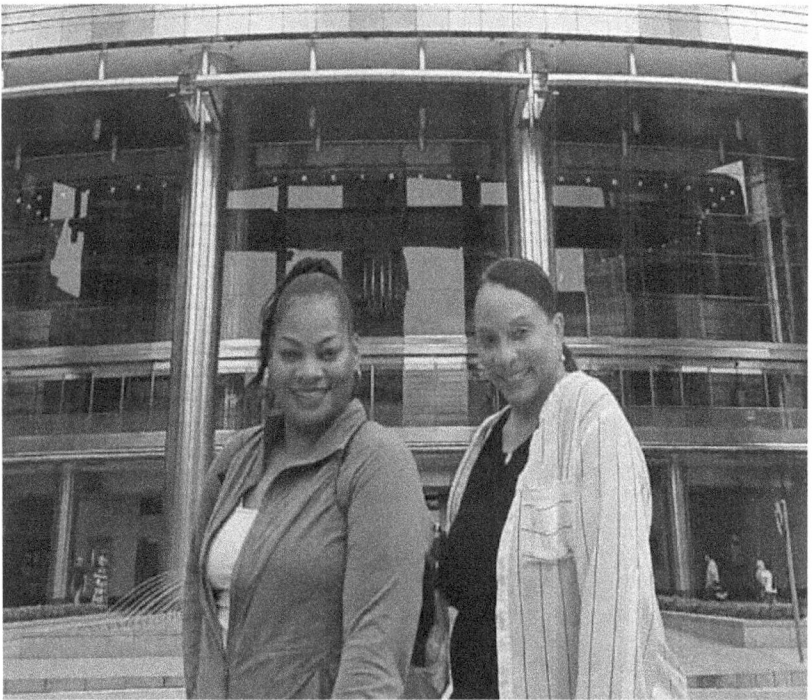

T-Que Winning & Dr. LaJoyce at the stainless-steel Petronas Twin Towers in Kuala Lumpur, Malaysia — the tallest twin towers in the world. (Photo Credit: Low Yee Ming)

CHAPTER 1

THE CURE FOR DISEASE IS PREVENTION

*"Beloved, I Pray that you may prosper in all things and be in
health, even as your soul prospers."*
–3 John 1:2

*"The most powerful medicine of all, is to teach people
how NOT to need it."*
–Hippocrates 360 B.C.

L et me be perfectly clear: disease is not a mystery. And the cure
for disease is not found in a pill bottle. The cure for disease is
Prevention. I cannot remain silent while the new face of Cancer is
getting younger and younger while people are dying from diseases
we can prevent.

Back in the days before Christ, Hippocrates was teaching this
simple truth that healers should be teaching people how NOT to
need medicine. This is a powerful sentiment which still stands
today.

It may not be a popular truth, but it is a spiritual and physiological
fact. Prevention is the act of *not* getting sick in the first place. And

1

the first step toward prevention is cleansing the body so that it may operate as the Divine machine it was designed to be.

When I speak of detoxing, I speak of returning to God's original blueprint, where our bodies are energized by living water, nourished by real food, and strengthened by daily motion, rest, and prayer. Where the temple is kept clean. Where we go Back to Eden... because if we don't, we soon will glow in the dark.

So many people today are surviving and not *thriving*. They are drinking caffeine to wake up, taking sleeping aids to fall asleep, using antacids to kill the burn of the bad food they cannot digest, and praying that the diseases of Mama, Daddy, and their Grandparents don't kill them. This is not health. This is bondage. Until it is understood that "Your Biography is NOT Your Biology," the goal of attaining Perfect Health will remain a wish.

And I know this bondage well. I have lived it. I have counseled it. I have wept with it. I share my personal story here because I am truly concerned about the fragile state of the health in this world. COVID showed us all our fragility and the question I ask today is, *Can your immunity conquer the next 'Goliath'?* It is important to keep the Immune System strong to be prepared for whatever may come your way.

Why am I so passionate about this? Because I am a woman who was married to a man who knew he had full-blown AIDS and did not tell me. Two years into the marriage—it's funny—he never mentioned it. (Read full account in *Faith Under Fire: Betrayed By A Thing Called Love)*. I thank God that I am HIV-negative thanks to being covered by The Blood of Jesus and having a rock-solid immune system. That stressful life event I mentioned earlier which led me to the Detox was learning my Prince Charming had AIDS. The Bronchial infection I could not shake, was the grief which settled in my lungs over learning I would become a young widow. Here is the good news: the body is brilliant! The body is resilient. And the body is wired to heal. If we simply *stop* interrupting its Divine processes with toxins, trauma, and triggers, it will do what it is already programmed to do.

10 Signs Your Body Needs a Detox:

1. Constantly feel fatigued, stressed, anxious, and overwhelmed.

2. Experience headaches and/or lack of mental clarity.

3. Easily catch Cold, Flu, Infections, and Viruses and often on medication.

4. Have an allergic response to the change of seasons with scratching, sneezing, itching, and wheezing that seems to calm with Antihistamines.

5. Carrying excess body weight or unable to gain weight.

6. Constipation is constant and uncomfortable because digestion is troublesome.

7. Often have skin breakouts and blemishes and/or a tired, dull, and lack-luster complexion.

8. Frequently have coffee, soda, alcohol, cigarettes, drugs

(prescription or otherwise).

9. Frequently slip into making less-healthy food choices often having fried foods, processed meat, processed foods, dairy, gluten, refined white sugar, fake sugar, and fast food.

10. Often being exposed to common environmental toxins such as carbon emissions, Second-hand or Third-hand smoke, herbicides, pesticides, artificial fragrances, and traditional household chemicals.

TRINITY is not just a program; it is a return. A return to balance. A return to clarity. A return to discipline. A return to honoring our bodies as sacred vessels.

This chapter is your foundation. Consider it your Wellness Wake-Up call and your Wellness contract. As you embark upon this 21-day journey, remember that the true cure for any disease lies within the power of *Prevention*.

Let us begin.

CHAPTER 2

ARE YOU WELLNESS ADJACENT?

*"Do you not know that your bodies are
temples of the Holy Spirit...?"*
−1 Corinthians 6:19-20

Many people talk about wanting to be healthy. They buy the vitamins. They scroll the wellness blogs. They like the fitness posts. They even join the gym. But when it comes time to act, they hesitate. They circle the runway. They walk on the outside of the fence. They stay "wellness adjacent."

Being wellness adjacent means you are near the truth, but not applying it. You know better, but do not *yet* do better. You desire change but fear the cost. I always say, *You can pay now or pay later, but one day, you **will** pay.* It is interesting how we spend the first half of our lives attaining wealth and then spend the second half of our lives spending that wealth to attain health. And I understand. I have seen this pattern in patients who cry during our consultations because they know exactly what they need to do, but feel paralyzed by the idea of letting go of those habits AND those stories that comfort them. Here is what I need you to know: discomfort is not your enemy. Disease is. Dis-Ease is absolutely your enemy. No matter what your faith background may be, every Holy book speaks of avoiding disease and staying well as a premise of their faith and maintaining good health. Each sacred tradition recognizes **health as a Divine gift**, a moral responsibility, and a spiritual pathway. Whether it is through prayer, food discipline, compassion, or detoxification, Wellness is spoken of in priority across all Holy texts:

1. The Bible: The Christian Tradition
"Beloved, I pray that you may prosper in all things and
be in health, just as your soul prospers."
~ 3 John 1:2 (NKJV)

This well-known verse explicitly links prosperity, wellness, and the soul. It underscores that God's desire is for us to flourish, not just spiritually, but also physically and emotionally.

2. The Quran: Islamic Tradition
"Eat of the good things We have provided for
your sustenance, but commit no excess therein."
~Surah Taha (20:81)

This verse encourages moderation to choose wholesome foods which are key elements of maintaining good health.

3. **The Tripitaka: Buddhist Tradition**
   "Health is the greatest gift, contentment the greatest wealth, faithfulness the best relationship."
   ~Dhammapada 204
   The Buddha elevated health as the **"greatest gift"**— higher even than material wealth. This reflects Buddhism's reverence for physical and mental well-being as a foundation for spiritual development.

4. **The Vedas: Hindu Tradition**
   "May all be happy. May all be free from illness. May all see what is auspicious. May no one suffer."
   ~Bṛhadāraṇyaka Upaniṣad 1.4.14
   (part of the Yajur Veda)

This verse, often recited as a peace invocation, is a prayer for the wellness of **all beings** and not just individuals, but communities and all of creation.

Also, from the Atharva Veda:
   "Let me receive medicine, the best and most potent, that brings wellness and long life."
   ~Atharva Veda 8.7.10

The Vedas honor herbs, breath, fasting, and seasonal cleansing. The ancient roots of natural healing are still honored in Ayurveda today.

The real cost of being wellness adjacent is not in choosing kale over cake or sleep over screens. The real cost is in the abandonment of what is sacred, co-pays, missed milestones, and days or experiences lost to doctor visits, chronic pain, and pills that put a Band-Aid over the bullet hole rather than cure the cause.

Your body is not a burden. It is a blueprint. A magnificent, miraculous vessel entrusted to you. It deserves your care, your attention, and your discipline.

So, I ask you now: Are you ready to step out of the shadows of being wellness adjacent and into the light of transformation? Will you stop dating wellness? The many people have placed wellness aside because they believed it cost too much to stay well are now spending money in the second half of their lives to attain health.. If this statement is a Wellness Wake-Up alarm for you, I ask…Are you finally ready to commit to fully *Becoming HealthyWealthy*?

Let us move forward.

CHAPTER 3

DETOX DEFINED: What It Is, What It Is Not

You shall know the truth, and the truth shall
make you free.
–John 8:32

The truth is that most people are carrying around years—yes, years—of accumulated waste inside their bodies. Many are weighed down by toxic residue embedded in their tissues, emotions they have never processed, and spiritual burdens that block Divine flow. They wonder why they feel sluggish, stuck, sick, and tired.

Let us get something straight. Detoxing is not a trend. It is not a juice fast for the sake of vanity, nor bragging rights. It is not a deprivation ritual, nor is it a punishment for poor food choices. Detoxing is a *Divine Recalibration.*

A Detox is defined as a short-term, intentional interruption of the body's toxic load so that it may reset, restore, and *return* to the way God designed it to function. It is a chance for the body's self-cleansing processes already coded into your DNA to activate and work without interference.

Make no mistake, the modern body is overwhelmed. From the air we breathe to the products we apply to our skin, from the processed foods on our plates, to the stress hormones surging through our bloodstream, we are burdened by invisible toxins daily. Over time, these toxins clog the Lymphatic system, congest the Liver, weaken the immune response, disrupt digestion, cloud the mind, and create a breeding ground for chronic disease.

That is why a Detox is necessary. And that is why the TRINITY Detox is different.

It is **not** a starvation protocol or a quick fix. It is a holistic process that addresses the physical, emotional, and spiritual root causes of toxicity. It provides the body with exactly what it needs to do what it was already created to do; cleanse itself.

Through TRINITY, you will nourish the body with two types of GOOD GREENS, and flush the system with hydration; purge Parasites with GOOD RIDDANCE; and have daily eliminations (I call them Evacuations) with GOOD & CLEAN COLON . You will support the Liver, calm the nervous system, and lighten the burden on every organ of elimination: skin, kidneys, lungs, lymph, and bowels.

And perhaps for the first time, you will *listen* to your body and respond with compassion, rather than attempting to silence its cries with temporary fixes, pills, caffeine, or self-blame.

You will also rest, Deeply.

You will hydrate, Intentionally.

You will move, Joyfully.

You will pray, Daily.

You will reclaim what belongs to you:

> Your Vitality.
>
> Your Clarity.
>
> Your Perfect Health.

So let us begin this journey of definition and distinction, where Detox is no longer a buzzword, but a sacred, life-affirming act of obedience and self-love.

CHAPTER 4

THE PARASITE PROBLEM: A HIDDEN BURDEN

*"And I will restore to you the years that the
cankerworm has eaten..."*
—Joel 2:25

Most people are walking around with **uninvited guests** living rent-free in their bodies. These guests do not knock, they do not ask permission, and they certainly do not clean up after themselves. They are **Parasites**. They thrive in darkness, in warm and sticky places, and in silence. You my friend, are the warm and sticky host the Parasites just love!

Parasites are the *silent saboteurs* of health. They hide in the intestines, muscle tissue, organs, and even the brain. They rob the body of nutrients. They inflame the gut. They release toxic waste. And they cause cravings - not for healthy foods - but for sugar, starch, and red meat, because these cravings are their foods, not yours.

And yet, most conventional medical systems are **silent** on the matter. Rarely are Parasites even considered in a diagnosis unless one has recently traveled to a Third World country. The truth?

Parasites are everywhere. In our food, water, soil, pets, and yes, even in our bodies.

Here is the scientific bona fide truth...I want to present a powerful visual which dismantles the myth that Parasites are rare or "only in some people". Every single one of us is full of microscopic "bugs" which are bacteria, fungi, and Parasites that live in the gut and overflow into the organs and the blood. While we are alive, with a healthy lifestyle, diet, and seasonal deworming programs, our immune system keeps the 'good bugs' in check and in their place. At the moment life leaves the body, the barriers are gone. No heartbeat. No circulation. No immune defense. And those bugs? They do what bugs do best; they spread.

Within a day or two of a dead body not being attended to in a timely fashion, the bacteria in the intestines multiply and begin traveling through the body. As gases build up, the pressure pushes them out of the gut and from other hiding places into the rest of the tissues. Soon, they begin moving outside of the body through every available opening.

When a body is left unattended after death, the Parasites and microbes begin *crawling out*. They are never crawling in.

This proves a critical point: they were already there, living inside us all along! They are not invaders waiting to sneak in after death because they want to feed on AND feed from living hosts. They are the quiet, hidden residents we carry throughout our lifetime causing people many health challenges.

How do you know if you have Parasites and need to deworm? You do not need a lab test to know. You need **truth**, discernment, and attention to your symptoms. I credit my mentor Dr. Frederick

Douglas Burton, my personal Medical Doctor and Alternative Therapy Doctor with an exquisite, foundational Parasite education. He taught me these simple truths that I have utilized clinically for more than 20 years.

Ask and answer these questions:

- Do you have seasonal allergies?

- Do you grind your teeth at night?

- Do you have itching around the rectum, nose, eyes, or ears?

- Do you crave sugar or red meat obsessively?

- Do you feel bloated, especially after eating fruit?

- Are you tired no matter how much you sleep?

- Do you have skin breakouts that will not clear?

- Do you have chronic skin conditions Rosacea, Eczema, Psoriasis, or acne?

- Do you have chronic constipation or any form of Irritable Bowel Disorder?

- Are you constantly coughing up phlegm or blowing your nose?

If you said yes to any of the above, Parasites may be at play.

The NIH reports that 70% of the global population lives with Parasites and don't even know it. According to their recent report on the impact of Parasites, *"Globally, annual death rates have increased from 200.000 in 2021 to over 700,000 reported deaths in 2025."*

These statistics are staggering. This is war. It's either you, or them. **Warfare Requires a Weapon** to win this battle, because we are outnumbered.

The TRINITY Detox includes **GOOD RIDDANCE** for this very reason. It is our **biological eviction notice** to the Parasites. With herbs that have been used for centuries—Black Walnut, Clove, Wormwood, Garlic, and Aloe Vera—we declare war on these freeloaders.

You cannot starve them.

You cannot wish them away.

You must draw them out to die.

When paired with GOOD & CLEAN COLON, which scrubs the intestines, GOOD RIDDANCE dislodges the Parasites from their hiding places. Then, the GOOD GREENS Formulas #1 & #2 with Spirulina and Chlorophyll work as blood purifiers, binders, and chelators to heal and restore what the Parasites have damaged.

This is **strategic warfare**, and it works.

What comes out will shock you. Yes, you will see them. Sometimes in clusters. Sometimes long and stringy. Sometimes as what looks like mucus or threads. Do not panic…**PRAISE!**

Because what you flush out is the very thing stealing your health.

It is better in the bowl than in your body.

It is better out than hidden and wreaking havoc.

My Mommie always said, "There is always more room out than in."

After the house is clean, it has to be kept in order, lest worse things return. Likewise, after Parasite removal, you must maintain a clean internal environment. That is why TRINITY is not just a cleanse, it is a reset and redirection. It brings you into alignment with God's design.

You were never meant to be a host to *anything* that depletes you.

Let us clean house and reclaim your Perfect Health.

CHAPTER 5

SOLID SOLUTIONS...POWERED BY NATURE

*"The leaves of the tree were for the
healing of the nations."*
–Revelation 22:2

In a world overflowing with synthetic answers and chemical fixes, TRINITY stands unapologetically as a return to what is *natural*, what is *pure*, and what is *powerful*. The products in TRINITY are Solid Solutions, Powered by Nature.

When I say "solid solutions," I am referring to the four formulas in the TRINITY Detox Program that work together synergistically to transform your body from the inside out: GOOD GREENS #1, GOOD GREENS #2, GOOD RIDDANCE, and GOOD & CLEAN COLON. These are not trendy powders or mystery drops. They are nature-sourced, time-tested tools crafted with clinical precision, and herbal wisdom.

GOOD GREENS FORMULA #1: 100% pure Hawaiian Spirulina. A potent blood cleanser, antioxidant, and cellular rebuilder. It detoxifies, energizes, and nourishes your cells with every dose to Alkalinize. Energize. Nourish.

GOOD GREENS FORMULA #2: Chlorophyll from White Mulberry Leaves. It alkalinizes the body, purifies the bloodstream, and restores internal balance. This is living water in capsule form. The combination of the Chlorophyll with the Spirulina serves as a powerful chelator which drags out heavy metals and binds all other toxicity being shaken loose from the body for easy removal.

GOOD RIDDANCE: The Parasite & Deworming Herbal Complex. This addition makes the detox protocol *comprehensive and credible*. It distinguishes TRINITY as **not just a cleanse** but a *true systemic detox* due to the Parasite removal component, which most people overlook.

GOOD RIDDANCE is a fierce botanical blend of Black Walnut Hull, Clove Flower, Wormwood Leaf, Garlic, and Aloe Vera. This is your eviction notice to the microscopic Parasites who deplete your health and hijack your healing.

"Don't continue to be a warm, sticky Host to Parasites... Hoist them with GOOD RIDDANCE!

GOOD & CLEAN COLON: A cleansing blend with Plant Fiber, Roselle Berry, Organic Oats, Garcinia Cambogia, and Inulin. It ensures the pathways of elimination remain open and clear. No more buildup, no more blockage, no more constipation. GOOD & CLEAN COLON goes beyond elimination. It ensures a complete evacuation. Together, these formulas are your wellness workhorses. They are not merely supplements, they are assignments. Each one has a job to do, and when taken as instructed, they unlock the body's God-given power to heal.

These Solid Solutions are more than product names; they represent a promise. When you give the body what it needs, it will reward you with what you desire: a complete Detoxification. One mistake many people make is doing only one part of the work. They might try a colon cleanse, but forget that the blood is still dirty. They might take supplements but leave sludge in the intestines. Or they fast, but fail to replenish.

This is why the TRINITY Protocol is so effective. It honors the truth that healing happens best when the whole being is engaged.

EDMARK also gives the promise to source each product with the highest standards in the world. TRINITY is Halal, Non-GMO, GMP, Vegan, and with US FDA Standards.

Your body was divinely created to cleanse, regenerate, and repair itself. What it often lacks is support, a plan, a protocol, and a purpose. The good news is that no condition is permanent. That is why TRINITY works. It is a formula based on the threefold principle of healing the Body, Mind, and Spirit, together.

No More Buildup. No More Blockage. No More Constipation.

TRINITY is the solution for a problem many do not even know they have: internal congestion.

When you are blocked up physically, you are often blocked spiritually.

When your Bowels are sluggish, so is your motivation.

When your Liver is burdened, your mind is cloudy.

When your Lymphatic system is overloaded, your internal waste removal system becomes stagnant.

TRINITY brings the flow back.

Back to your gut.

Back to your bloodstream.

Back to your cells.

And back to your faith in knowing there is hope for your healing.

Because when people are sick and tired of being sick and tired, they will try almost anything. TRINITY is not just anything. It is everything you need to begin again.

Welcome to the garden. Welcome to TRINITY. Let the healing work of nature begin.

Chapter 6

The Emotional Unclogging

"Create in me a clean heart, O God; and renew a
right spirit within me."
–Psalm 51:10

O nce the colon clears and the Parasites are gone, something remarkable happens:

Your emotions begin to surface. Detoxing is not just physical. It is emotional.

The gut is often called the **"second brain"** for a reason because it stores tension, trauma, and unresolved emotion. When the bowels release, the emotions that were stuck there start to move too.

Many patients report unexpected waves of emotion during the TRINITY Detox:

- Sudden tears

- Old memories resurfacing

- Vivid dreams

- Unexplainable moments of peace

- Or even irritability followed by calm

This is normal.

This is necessary.

This is healing at the **Soul level.**

You may not remember the heartbreak from ten years ago, but your gut does.

You may not consciously relive the grief, betrayal, or circumstance, but it lives in the tissues. The same way trauma affects the heart and mind, it also affects the gut.

When you clean out the gut, you give the body permission to let go of what it has held onto. It is not just physical, but emotional.

The body cannot heal while holding grief. This is why I held onto a Bronchial infection for more than a month with the news of Prince Charming having AIDS.

The Liver cannot detox under the weight of rage.

The bowels cannot move freely while you are emotionally constipated. If you cannot swallow what has happened to you, digest it, and move on, other problems are on the horizon.

The Liver is where anger is held. As the Liver is cleansed, you may feel intense waves of anger. Some have reported feeling, *"as mean as a rattlesnake."*

Go ahead and write the letter you may never mail to the person who betrayed you.

Go ahead and pick up the phone to leave a message or voice text to 'let-them-have-it'.

Then go ahead and blame it on the Detox.

As these emotions come up, do not stifle the emotion. Swallowing what you really *want* or *need* to say causes other physiological symptoms that, if not dealt with, will cause you harm.

We do not fear tears during detox. We welcome them. Tears are the body's emotional elimination. Crying is not a breakdown. It is an emotional cleansing and a **BREAKTHROUGH**.

When the tears come ask yourself, *If these tears were words, what would they say?* If you feel heavy, journal.

If you feel angry, walk and breathe.

If you feel stuck, pray aloud.

If you feel hopeless, speak affirmations of life and promise.

Once the grief, clutter, and congestion leave, something beautiful moves in.

Joy. Hope. Clarity. Creativity, and Self-Love.

This period of Detoxification is the perfect time to:

- Disconnect from the news and digital devices.

- Release relationships that no longer serve you which leave you drained.

- Spend quiet time in prayer or Scripture.

- Speak life to your reflection in the mirror.

- Lighten your calendar to honor rest.

This is not selfish. This is sacred.

It is about creating space for the things that matter, and YOU matter. Saying NO gives you the opportunity to be more present with the things you have said YES to. Saying YES to a 21-day reset is a huge step toward a new beginning.

Let your gut speak.

Let your Spirit respond.

Let your heart be made clean again.

The Spirit of heaviness lifts. Your appetite changes. Your cravings shift. Your inner voice gets louder and it speaks truth. You will begin to be a reflection of the commitment to self.

No lies. No shame. No fear.

You feel more like yourself than you have in years. Because, in truth (see...truth keeps resurfacing), that version of you was never really gone. You have been buried beneath the buildup.

This is your emotional evacuation, and it is your right of divine passage toward becoming the Whol-istic person God created and becoming HealthyWealthy.

CHAPTER 7

THE HEALTHYWEALTHY LIFE BEGINS

"Let us cleanse ourselves from all filthiness of the flesh and spirit, perfecting holiness in the fear of God."
–2 Corinthians 7:1

HealthyWealthy defined is recognizing that the greatest fortune you can ever possess is the vitality to live fully, love deeply, and serve your purpose without being held hostage by poor health.

HealthyWealthy is the undeniable truth that health *is* wealth. It is the state of being where your body, mind, and Spirit are so well-nourished and well-functioning that they become your greatest assets.

- **It is freedom.** Freedom from pain, prescriptions, preventable disease, and the heavy costs of neglect.

- **It is abundance.** Abundance of energy, clarity, joy, and resilience that no money can buy.

- **It is sustainability.** When you invest in your health today, you are securing wealth for tomorrow because doctor bills, hospital stays, and lost years sometimes cost more than you can pay.

- **It is alignment.** To be HealthyWealthy is to live in sync with the natural laws of the body, where prevention is the cure and wellness is not a privilege but your birthright.

Now that the body has purged waste, released toxins, and evicted unwanted guests, it is time to rebuild the temple.

Just like a house that has been deep-cleaned and fumigated, the next step is to restore the structure by laying down new structure, replacing what was broken with clarity, and fortifying the foundation with nutrients.

Healing is not complete without Restoration. Cleansing clears the way, but replenishing keeps the way clear.

When the gut is clean, it is ready for the continuation of healthy microbes.

Though TRINITY includes the prebiotic **Inulin**, it is the ideal time to include:

- Probiotics with fermented foods like sauerkraut, kimchi, organic yogurt, or kombucha

- Hydration with clean water and herbal teas

- Fresh fruits and vegetables

A healthy gut is a healthy brain, a healthy mood, and a strong immune system. Rebuilding it is essential for long-term success.

When you continue to pour living water and nourishing greens into your system after cleansing, it is not just health, it is an opportunity to honor God by taking care of the body He designed. You are restoring the years toxins stole your energy, Parasites clouded your clarity, and processed food robbed your waistline and pertinent health markers.

This is where your **HealthyWealthy Life** begins.

Restoration leads to:

- Radiant skin
- Peaceful sleep
- Focused thought
- Renewed drive
- Balanced blood sugar and blood pressure
- And yes, Joy

This is when people around you start asking what you are doing. This is when your pants fit differently. This is when you wake up without groaning. This is when you smile without trying.

You have flushed the old and fed the new.

You have cleansed the body, activated cellular repair, and added life to your years.

You are not just feeling better.

You are becoming better.

The question now becomes:

How do you stay clean and clear?

It is one thing to detox. It is another to live in a perpetual state of detoxification. While TRINITY is designed to be completed at the change of every season, GOOD GREENS FORMULAS #1 & #2 should be taken daily (see TRINITY DETAILS).

If you don't think you need to stay in a state of detoxification, just consider how many times a day your senses are assaulted by just breathing. Walking into a freshly mopped building wreaking of bleach or another cleaning agent that makes you choke and your eyes water. Or, even walking down the grocery store aisle where the cleansing products are sold. The out-gasses from those products in what I call the 'chemical aisle', are to be avoided if you don't want to inhale toxic burden. Not to mention fighting through smokers in doorways to get to your destination. So, you see, it is not as easy as you think to avoid daily assaults to your immune system. It happens more times per day than you realize.

This makes a good case for clean living to be a lifestyle goal. Detoxing once and returning to toxic habits is like detailing a car and then driving it through mud the next day. You were not simply detoxing for weight loss or energy. You were detoxing to improve your life and to increase your longevity.

The TRINITY Protocol is more than a 21-day cleanse. It is an introduction to a new way of being what is cleaner, clearer, and calmer.

To stay clean and clear:

- Choose whole foods that come from the earth, not a box, or a drive-thru.

- Stay hydrated with clean water daily.

- Eat with intention, not emotion.

- Fast occasionally to give your organs rest.

- Move your body to pump the blood and lymph.

- Protect your Peace like it is sacred…because it is. To quote my dear friend, Dr. Sheri Riley, "Peace is the new Success." Indeed it is!

The detox helps reset your internal terrain to an alkaline state where disease cannot survive. To maintain that environment:

- Avoid excess sugar, dairy, red meat, and processed food.
- Continue with greens, lemon water, raw vegetables, and sea vegetables.
- Include herbs and minerals to minimize oxidative stress to your cells.
- Maintain bowel regularity. DO NOT GET CONSTIPATED.

A clean colon and alkaline system create conditions where inflammation, viruses, and cancer cells **cannot thrive**.

Keeping a clear mind is imperative! Toxic thoughts lead to toxic behaviors. Toxic behaviors lead to toxic results. The same way you flushed your colon, you must also detox your thoughts, and sometimes, purge that Contacts list.

Daily renewal comes from:

- Scripture and prayer
- Gratitude journaling
- Silence and solitude
- Limiting digital input
- Protecting your eye gates, ear gates, and the heart

You have already made space. Now it is time to fill that space wisely.

This is your new Normal. Do not fear returning to the old ways. You are not the same. You have new awareness, new tools, and a new connection with your body and Spirit. And now that you know what it feels like to be clean, clear, and free.

You will never again confuse feeling poorly as **normal**.

Let your new normal be one of:

- Consistent elimination

- Balanced moods

- Clear thinking

- Deep rest

- Unapologetic Discipline

What does it look like to be HealthyWealthy?

A well body makes well decisions.

A clear mind attracts Divine strategy.

A nourished system has the stamina to fulfill its purpose.

You cannot serve fully while sick.

You cannot pour out when you are depleted.

You cannot break generational curses with generational diseases.

This is why TRINITY is not a trend. It is a **transformational foundation**.

When you are well, you:

- You are no longer surviving. You are **thriving**.

- Your body is lighter.

- Your mind is sharper.

- Your emotions are balanced. You have flushed the waste, healed your gut, evicted the Parasites, replenished your cells, and made peace with your past.

Now you can:

- Show up Shining.

- Parent with Patience.

- Create with Clarity.

- Build with Boldness.

- Age with Grace.

- And live without fear of a fateful future.

You are no longer chasing good health.

You are **living it.**

Maintenance Is Mastery of your body. At the change of every season, repeat the 21-Day TRINITY Detox, or more frequently if a health challenge persists.

And now, it is time to **build a life that reflects it.** When your body is clean, your mind is renewed, your Spirit is strong, and your decisions are aligned, you reflect the Kingdom of God on earth. That is the goal.

What are you reflecting? When your skin glows, your eyes brighten, and your waistline returns, people will ask what you are doing. When you no longer need caffeine to wake up or medication to fall asleep, people will want to know your secret.

Let your life be the testimony.

Let your lifestyle do the talking.

Because when others see your results, they will start to believe it is possible for them too.

TRINITY is not just about *detoxing* the body. It is about becoming a **HealthyWealthy** able bodied person capable of receiving, building, and being a good steward of the life God designed just for you.

The goal is not perfection.

The goal is alignment.

Stay tuned in. Stay in tune. You have become Healthy Wealthy.

CHAPTER 8

FAQs & CLINICAL OBSERVATIONS

"In all thy getting, get understanding."
–Proverbs 4:7

It is time to address what every person wonders next:
"Can I really do this?"
"What if I have health conditions?"
"What will it feel like?"
"What should I expect?"

This chapter answers the most frequently asked questions from those considering the TRINITY Detox, as well as insights gathered through years of clinical observation and the patient experience.

Frequently Asked Questions

Q: What day should I begin the detox?
A: You may begin the detox on any day you choose. The calendar only has numbered days for this reason. Many report that they like beginning mid-week because the first couple of days are

nourishment before the cleanses begin. Start whenever it is most convenient.

Q: What is the most important thing to do before getting started?
A: Getting organized is the BEST thing to do first. Read all of the labels and know the quantities of each product you will take. Many people have reported being so excited to begin that they took only one of everything on the first day. This is incorrect. PLEASE READ the instructions first.

Q: What can help me to feel ready to get started?
A: Going grocery shopping for the items you need to help ensure maximum results will allow you to have all you need at home to make meals. It will be labor intensive if the clean food is not readily available. This also fosters poor choices when you're starving because the drive-thru is always available. Keep the good choices handy.

Q: After reading all of the instructions and grocery shopping, I feel overwhelmed. Help!
A: I understand the feeling! Take the instructions day-by-day. Do not look ahead more than 1-2 days for what is coming next, or yes, the sense of being overwhelmed will definitely take over. Detox success = Determination + Discipline. You've got this!

Q: Due to my work schedule, I am sleeping at 3pm when the instructions say I should have finished the GOOD GREENS by 3pm. What should I do? And what about the other products too?

A: Here are the general rules to follow:

- Always take GOOD RIDDANCE on an empty stomach before a meal.

- Take the GOOD GREENS Formulas any time after waking because they are energy boosters. Taking the GOOD GREENS Formulas too late in the day or less than 6-7 hours before bedtime may prohibit you from sleeping.

- Always take GOOD & CLEAN COLON after dinner with 1-2 glasses of water.

Q: I don't like to use the bathroom in public places. Will I be going to the bathroom a lot?
A: Yes, the bathroom...any bathroom needs to become your friend. Please, PLEASE do NOT suppress the urge to pee or poop - yes, even in public places. Holding the urge to eliminate is one of the fastest ways to disease. The body is detoxing, which means it is expelling toxicity through the eliminative organs.

Q: We get in trouble at my job for going to the bathroom too often. How can I complete the detox?
A: This is an awful violation of your rights to health! The Occupational Safety and Health Administration (OSHA) has this to say about your concern: *"An employer can be in violation of an OSHA regulation if they restrict employees from using the bathroom frequently. OSHA requires employers to allow workers to leave their work to use the restroom when needed and prohibits unreasonable restrictions on use. The goal of OSHA's sanitation*

standard is to prevent adverse health effects and ensure workers can promptly use toilet facilities when necessary."
Enough said.

Q: Can I do TRINITY if I am on medication?
A: Yes. In most cases, TRINITY can be used safely alongside prescribed medications. However, medications should be taken at least 1 hour apart from detox products. Always consult your health provider and monitor for changes in how your body responds. You may notice you need *less* medication as your system detoxes. Monitor your numbers and keep a log.

Q: What if I do not have a Gallbladder?
A: You can still do the TRINITY Detox. If you do not have a Gallbladder there is extra burden being placed upon the Liver. This program will be a welcome cleansing.

Q: Is this safe during pregnancy or breastfeeding?
A: NO. Detoxification during pregnancy or lactation is **not advised**, as toxins being released could enter the baby's bloodstream or breast milk. Wait until after delivery and weaning before beginning TRINITY. However, **Good Greens #1 (Spirulina)** and **Good Greens #2 (Chlorophyll)** can be taken as maintenance doses only during pregnancy and lactation:

- Take **4 Good Greens #1 (Spirulina)** tablets

- Add **1 capsule of Good Greens #2 (Chlorophyll)** to **32 oz of water daily and drink throughout the day**

This provides gentle nourishment without triggering a detoxification effect.

Q: Will I need to be near a bathroom all day?
A: No. Most eliminations occur predictably within 6 to 12 hours of taking Good & Clean Colon. It is best taken in the evening. After a couple of days, you will be able to adjust to your body's natural rhythm as to what time is best before the elimination process begins.

Q: Is TRINITY safe for children?
A: Absolutely!
- Ages 13-17 should use half of all quantities recommended.
- Ages 10-12 should use only when under the care of a Qualified Holistic Healthcare Practitioner.

Q: Can I continue exercising while detoxing?
A: Yes, and exercise is encouraged. I don't recommend a marathon or heavy weightlifting during this time. But gentle movement like walking, stretching, rebounding, and lymphatic massage can support faster results. However, strenuous exercise may feel tiring in the first few days. Listen to your body.

Q: What can I eat during the 21 days?
A: While TRINITY does not require fasting or a strict diet, eating **clean and alkaline** foods will enhance results. Emphasize fruits, vegetables, herbal teas, whole grains, organic chicken or turkey, and wild-caught fish. Avoid sugar, alcohol, dairy, and processed foods. **PLEASE NOTE: Do not fast during the 21-days.**

Q: I need to do a Detox but I don't want to lose weight?
A: It is important to understand that toxicity holds on to waste. Just because you do not want to lose weight does not mean you are in optimum health. Once the waste has been eliminated from the body, you will be able to maintain a healthy weight. You may be holding on to more waste than you realize. Allow nature to do the work and take-out the guesswork about the toxicity level in your body.

Q: I have tried detoxing previously and it did not work?
A: Detoxifying the body and being on a Wellness Journey is not a sprint, it is a marathon. Give yourself some time and grace to build the life you want. Change will take time and be well worth it.

Q: How often should I complete the 21-Day Detox?
A: TRINITY should be completed at the change of every season because this is the time Parasites are having more babies inside of you who deposit waste resulting in an accumulation of Candida contributing to seasonal allergies, and skin issues to name a few.

- The Detox can also be completed anytime negative symptoms are compromising your quality of life.

- In cases of a chronic illness, more frequent use may be utilized but only under the care of a Qualified Healthcare Practitioner.

- **GOOD GREENS** Formulas #1 and #2 can be taken as daily supplementation independently when not engaging in the full 21-Day Detox.

Q: What should I eat during the Detox for the best results?
A: When eating, consider the rainbow, and ask yourself, *Is this a clean food?*

- Vegetables

- Fruit

- Smoothies

- Fresh Squeezed Juice

- Wild-Caught Fish

- Organic Chicken

- Turkey

- Baked Sweet Potatoes or Baked/Roasted White Potatoes

- Hummus/Guacamole/Organic Tortilla Chips/ Salsa

- Organic Yogurt

- Fresh Popped Organic Popcorn

- Nuts

- Organic Cane Sugar, Maple Syrup, Honey, Stevia, Monk Fruit, or Coconut Sugar

- Quinoa, Black Rice, Sprouted Bread, and Unbleached flour

THE NO-NO LIST TO AVOID

- White Sugar & Sugar Substitutes (it feeds the Parasites you are eliminating!)

- Artificial Sweeteners (deposit acid crystals)

- White Rice, White Bread, White Pasta, Bleached Flour, Wheat Bread Pasteurized Cow Milk (all create a warm, sticky and yeast environment in the gut for Parasites to flourish)

- Beef/Pork/Organ Meat/Ox Tails/Goat (all contain Uric Acid)

- Soda

- Alcohol

- Coffee, Black/White/Green Tea or any caffeine products (these deposit acid residue -vs-Alkalinity)

- Energy Drinks

- Frozen Vegetables

- Canned Food

- Vegetable Oil

- Canola Oil

- Fast Food

Q: What should I drink during the Detox?

A: Hydration with water is necessary to flush toxins away. Drink up!

- Drink Half your body weight in ounces of water w/ Lemon. (for example, if weight=200 pounds, drink 100oz water per day)

- Dissolve or open 1 capsule of **GOOD GREENS #2 Chlorophyll** in a 16.8oz bottle of water before 3pm (I like to drink it all at once with the **GOOD GREENS #1 SPIRULINA as this intensifies the Detoxifying effect.**)

- Herbal Teas

- Fruit or Vegetable Smoothies

- Fruit or Vegetable Juice

- Sparingly - Organic Raw Milk, Almond, or Oat Milk

- Avoid Alcohol

- Avoid Soda

- Avoid Caffeine

Q: WHAT CAN I EXPECT DURING THE DETOX?

A: Here are just a few things to expect and To Do:

- Many Parasites and Worms are microscopic in nature, but you may purge Parasites or Worms that are visible. If seeing these in the toilet makes you squeamish, just wipe and flush!

- Mouth will have a green tint if GOOD GREENS FORMULA #1 is chewed. If you are unable to brush your teeth or eat following chewing, simply swallow or dissolve the tablets.

- Due to the Chlorophyll density of GOOD GREENS FORMULA #2, Drink with a straw if you are unable to brush or eat following drinking (This fact makes a good case for drinking all at once!)

- Also…due to the Chlorophyll density, urine may have a green-ish tint and bowel eliminations WILL be green.

- Will have more eliminations than usual, so use a plant-based wipe to avoid a sore rectum.

- Will urinate more frequently as the body is cleansing.

- May feel more fatigued than usual or have Cold/Flu-like symptoms. This is the detoxification process at work.

- **Go to bed by 10pm** in a dark room to help the body heal.

- May experience anal and body itching.

- Breath may be foul, be certain to brush teeth 3x per day and floss at least1x per day with a fluoride-free toothpaste and use an herbal mouthwash.

- Tongue may be coated white. This is a sign that toxicity is leaving the body. Be certain to brush your tongue, cheeks, roof of mouth, and crevices as Parasites love to hide in a warm mouth. Use a new toothbrush weekly.

- Use a wet washcloth or a wet paper towel to clean your nose. There will be an accumulation of mucus in your nose daily and it may itch. Using a Neti Pot is an excellent cleansing tool and can help fully flush the nasal cavity.

- There will be additional accumulated crusted mucus in eyes.

- Bathe or shower EVERY DAY before bed. The skin is the largest eliminative organ and toxins are being excreted daily. Additionally, you get 3 million new skin cells daily.

- Use an exfoliating cloth, gloves, or loofah to help slough-off the dead skin cells with an all-natural soap.

- Use a clean towel daily. All of the dead skin cells are on the towel.

- Experience optimum energy by exercising for at least 20 minutes per day.

- It is HIGHLY encouraged for couples to complete the program simultaneously because they may pass Parasites one to another.

- Monitor Blood Pressure and Sugar levels daily. Individuals have reported a decrease in their numbers while on the program.

- If you miss a day, get back on track. If you fall down with one of the items to avoid…Get back up!

WHAT ARE SOME OF THE POTENTIAL BENEFITS FROM THE SIDE-EFFECTS?

- As the body eliminates toxic waste you may have bouts of discomfort which should pass as the stubborn toxins leave the body.

- May cough-up phlegm due to the release of waste. **DO NOT SWALLOW** the phlegm! Do not be alarmed at the color or smell. This is old toxicity being expelled.

- Will have an accumulation of eye gunk, ear crust and wax, dried mucus in nose, and smelly under arms.

- Crying spells—as toxins leave the body, so do old and negative emotions leave.

- May finally get the courage to write someone the letter to whom you need to say goodbye…Or…the courage to write the letter to just to purge your feelings that you may never mail.

CLINICAL OBSERVATIONS

With over two decades of using this protocol, I have observed:

- The reluctancy to commit to detoxing and being grateful they did.

- Some patients release **1 to 3 feet of old waste** within the first day.

- Parasites are often expelled without the user realizing it and is sometimes mistaken for mucus or undigested food.

- Emotional releases are **common and welcome**: crying, irritability, fatigue, or vivid dreams.

- **Skin clears up** rapidly by week two.

- **Weight loss** is often noticeable by week one, but the more powerful result is the **feeling of lightness and energy.**

- Long-standing symptoms like **joint pain, brain fog, gas, bloating, and menstrual imbalance** often subside or vanish.

- Patients with **diabetes or high blood pressure** often report needing to adjust or reduce medication under medical supervision.

TRINITY works because it addresses the **root**, not just the symptoms.

CHAPTER 9

TESTIMONY TIME:
IF I GAVE YOUR BODY THE MIC,
WHAT WOULD IT SAY?

REAL TALK. REAL PEOPLE.
REAL HEALTH PRAISE REPORTS.
SUCCESS STORIES FROM AROUND THE WORLD

"I will tell of your goodness: all day long I will speak of your salvation, though it is more than I can understand."
–Psalm 71:15-16

If I gave my body The Mic today, it would say, "Thank you for the discipline." I was once known as the little freak who ate mainly vegetables. I quit pork and beef in high school. I carried around water bottles before hydration was trendy, and I endured relentless teasing for my choices. My friends made fun of me because I always wanted to leave the parties early. But the truth was, I was sleepy. Just genuinely tired by 9 o'clock, and I still am today!

My parents understood. They drove me to events knowing my exit time was not about curfew, it was about listening to my body.

Those early lifestyle habits became my salvation. They were the **"Stay ready so you do not have to get ready"** choices that strengthened my immune system and protected my health. I had no idea back then that my discipline would be the very thing that would be a contributing factor in saving my life.

Years later, the man I married called me *Rabbit* because of my healthy eating habits and my commitment to rest.

What I did not know was that those habits would become a shield.

A fortress.

A covering.

Because it was the same discipline that protected me from his HIV status. So, let me say it louder for the people in the back... If I gave my body The Mic today, it would say, "LaJoyce, Thank you for the DISCIPLINE!"

Now, here is your Wellness Wake-up. Honestly answer the question: If I gave *your* body The Mic, what would it say?

Would it say:

- "Please give me water."

- "No more parties this week."

- "I need sleep."

- "I want a good meal."

- "I do not want another soda!"

- "I have not had a bowel movement in days."

- "I need to stop smoking."

- "I need to detox."

Poor habits can be broken. All you have to do is stop investing in poor habits, turn around and walk in the opposite direction. Some say, it sounds simple. Walking in the other direction begins with a decision maintained by discipline.

You now have language and experience. You have walked through the protocol and seen what is possible.

Use it to teach your children.

Use it to care for your parents.

Use it to empower your Village.

Use it to interrupt generational patterns of sickness and poor nutrition.

Use it to glorify God in your body.

You do not have to be a doctor to make an impact.

You just need to share what worked.

Your story has power.

That said, it's Testimony Time! Here is Real Talk, from Real People, with Real Health Praise Reports from around the world who are choosing to take The Mic about their TRINITY Detox experience:

"This is my day 17 on the Detox plan and I have lost 7 pounds! My face looks brighter, and my skin is smoother. I feel more energetic and clear-minded."
~*Eileen A.—Delaware*~

"This extremely important information brought forth with the Detox has given me the health success I know is in Divine Order. I highly recommend this health regimen!"
~*Bishop Williams—New York*~

"When I started my first day of Trinity, I was curious about what it could do. At first, not much changed until day 4! I felt extra thirsty, my skin was dry, and I had mild cramps. But after 7 days, WOW—what a difference! I felt lighter, more energetic, and super focused at work. My skin looked clearer, and even during my period, I had zero usual PMS symptoms!"
~Reena J.—Phillipines~

"I decided to put the Detox advice into action. I started drinking kale and beets and exercising 3 times a week and I lost over 50 pounds. My Blood Pressure is now 117/74 and it has been the same for several days. I no longer need the pills! Thank you for helping me with this Detox program!"
~Lorenzo M.—North Carolina~

"The secrets to detoxifying are finally available in a way that fits into our everyday lives and hectic lifestyles—served up in a fashion that is just what The "Good" Doctor ordered."
~Karu D.—New York~

"I have struggled with seasonal allergies my whole life and I was depended on prescription and over-the-counter drugs to make my symptoms go away. I was a total skeptic about this program, but once I completed it, I am now a true believer!"
~Stephen E.—Georgia~

"I had no idea how toxic I was. I felt dead inside—emotionally, mentally, spiritually. TRINITY pulled me out of that pit. I

released what did not belong. I gained clarity, hope, energy, and peace. I don't just recommend it—I preach it."
~Rev. Thomas B.—Pennsylvania~

"TRINITY Provided me with a LOT energy, I lost a few pounds, my skin is supple, and my nails are strong."
~ Authur D.—Florida ~

"TRINITY is the real deal! I know my colon is real clean!"
~ Millicent B.—New Jersey ~

"On exactly my 14th day of taking Good Riddance I noticed big changes. It felt like there was a 'war' going on inside my tummy. My sleeping pattern completely shifted—I felt unusually sleepy throughout the day and I had very little appetite as if my stomach constantly felt full. Another major change was in my bowel movements. During the second week it increased from twice a day to four to five times daily. After every meal, I immediately had to rush to the toilet. It felt like my body was saying, "First in, first out!" By the third week that war was over. I felt lighter, enjoyed better sleep, and continued to have healthy and improved digestion. The program has made a huge difference in how I feel and I'm grateful for the positive changes it brought to my health."
~Archie V.—Phillipines~

"After the detox I felt energized and relaxed. I was regulated more than I have ever been. I wasn't bloated and I slept like a baby. The sleep was incredible"
~ *Andreé S. - Florida* ~

"After 21 days on TRINITY, I felt lighter, more energized, and no longer sluggish. My sleep schedule finally fell into place and I dropped 12 pounds. Total win for me!"
~ *MaryBeth A. - Georgia* ~

"TRINITY Provided me with a LOT energy, I lost a few pounds, my skin is supple, and my nails are strong."
~ *Authur D. – Florida* ~

"TRINITY is the real deal! I know my colon is real clean!"
~ *Millicent B. – New Jersey* ~

These are not exaggerations.

These are real people, with real lives, real pain, and real results. They are proof that when the body is supported, when the Spirit is nourished, and when the truth is embraced, **Healing Happens**.

Your Testimony is next. Whether your breakthrough is in your increased bowel frequency or your bloodwork, whether it is physical, emotional, or spiritual…**it counts**.

Share your story.

Document your journey.

Celebrate your milestones.

Someone else's healing may depend on your courage to step up to The Mic.

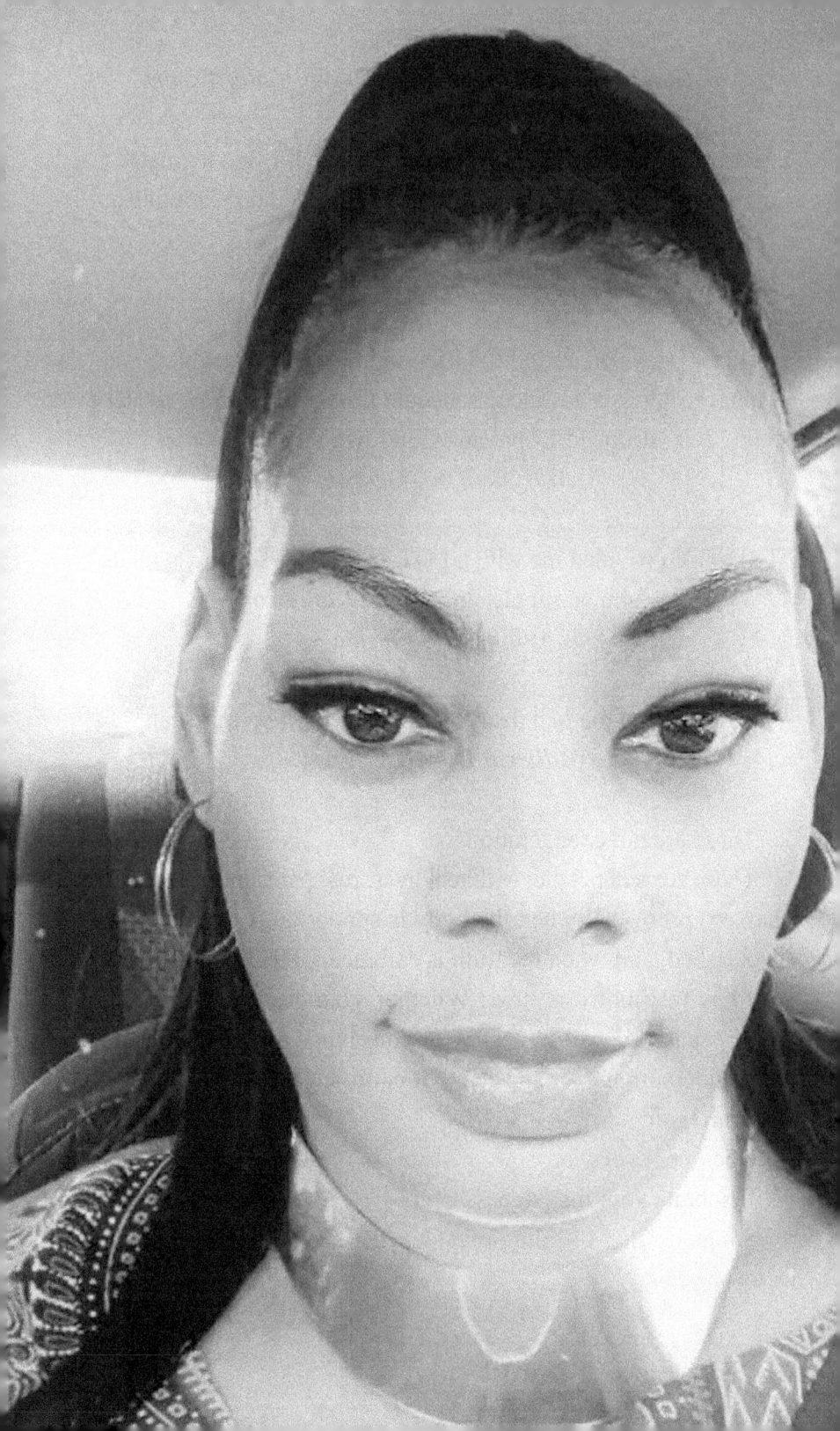

CHAPTER 10

A Final Word:
The Reset That Changed Everything
~ by ~
T-Que Winning

First, I want to acknowledge and honor my friend, Dr. LaJoyce Brookshire. It's one thing to dream, but it's another thing entirely to move on that dream—especially when the process is costly, complex, and spiritual. LaJoyce, thank you for being bold enough to walk it out. TRINITY isn't just a product, it's your legacy. And I'm honored to be part of the journey that brought it to life.

It all started with a phone call, but really, it began long before that.

We were at an EDMARK event in Baltimore, and I had invited Dr. LaJoyce and a few of my friends to come experience what EDMAK had to offer. By the time they tasted the products—especially the CoCollagen and the Ginseng Coffee—they were all buzzing with curiosity and excitement. But LaJoyce, being the holistic expert she is, wasn't just impressed. She was observing. She saw the energy in the room, heard the testimonies, but she also noticed something missing.

"There's nothing in this lineup that specifically targets parasites," she told me later. And that was a lightbulb moment.

She began looking deeper into some of the ingredients, and

while she respected the results people were getting, her spirit knew there was more. She saw an opportunity, not to compete, but to complete the mission. She wanted to present her own product line, one she had been building quietly in her heart for some time.

After the event, she called me and said, "T, I really want to speak with Chairman. I think there's a conversation to be had here." I asked her what she wanted me to say, and she started listing a few things to pass along. But I stopped her. "No, LaJoyce. You are the best person to pitch this. This is your baby. I'll give you his direct number. Call him yourself."

She did. And to no surprise, Chairman was intrigued. The two of them had a deep conversation on WhatsApp. Fast forward a few weeks, and in December 2024, she told me she had been invited to Malaysia to formally present her product line. And not only that, she asked me to go with her.

So, in January 2025, we packed our bags and flew across the world.

From the moment we landed, it felt like a divine appointment. We were picked up and greeted with the kind of warmth and honor that felt like a red carpet was being rolled out just for us. The twin towers gleamed in the distance, and we soaked in the beauty of Malaysia. But the real experience began when we arrived at Edmark Headquarters.

That building was pristine. Every floor looked untouched, even though it was clearly operating daily. We toured the packaging areas, watching the production lines for the CoCollagen, Bubble Tea, and Ginseng Coffee, and everything just radiated excellence. It was there, in that moment, that I knew something big was about to be birthed.

When we stepped into the conference room, I was so proud to sit beside Dr. LaJoyce. Watching her present TRINITY was like watching destiny walk into the room. She spoke with conviction, backed by science, experience, and purpose. Before the meeting began, she had all of us sign an NDA. Once everything was laid out on the table, the deal was sealed.

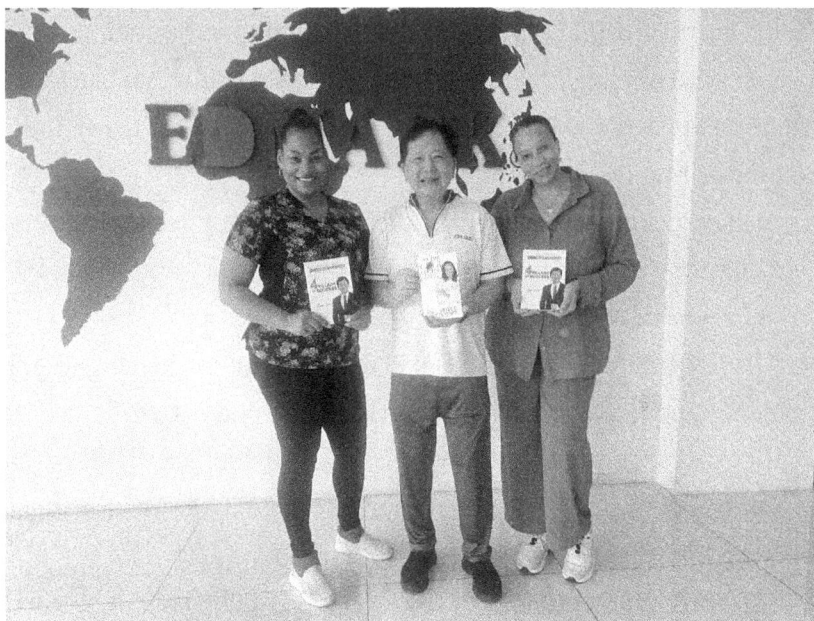

L to R: T-Que Winning, Chairman of EDMARK Mr. Sam Low, and Dr. LaJoyce Brookshire at the EDMARK International headquarters in Malaysia January 2025.

That night, we celebrated. We dined, we laughed, and we meditated on the magnitude of what had just happened. Something truly shifted in the spirit while we were there. Malaysia changed us. And what came next was history in the making.

The team wasted no time. Designs were drafted. Packaging was created. Edits were made. They went into full production. And soon, Trinity was born.

When TRINITY launched, I got one of the very first boxes.

Now let me be real with you. Yes, I work out. I eat clean most days. But there was one thing I couldn't shake. Key Lime Pie. Not just any kind—the Edwards brand, the one in the freezer section. I could finish a whole box in two days, no guilt, no hesitation.

But that craving? That was something else. I didn't realize I was fighting against something inside of me. And that's when Trinity started telling on me.

I started with Step One and increased my water intake. The very next day, I was in the bathroom. Not once. Not twice. But often. And I hadn't even moved past the first step yet.

By Day Three, my armpits had an odor that made me pause. I remembered LaJoyce saying that when your body starts detoxing, it'll push things out through your skin. And she was right. I was breaking out in small bumps. My appetite decreased. And the sugar cravings? Gone.

I wasn't hungry the way I used to be. My belly wasn't bloated. My body was purging—and it felt like it was finally breathing.

Doing TRINITY is like cleaning out your refrigerator.

You can't expect to bring in fresh fruits and vegetables and stack them on top of spoiled food and sticky shelves. You've got to throw away what's expired. You have to clean out the old leftovers, wipe down the stains, and sanitize the space.

Your gut is the refrigerator of your body. If you want a reset, you have to be honest with what's been sitting in there too long.

TRINITY doesn't play with you. And you shouldn't play with it either. If you're not going to do it fully, don't do it at all. Because once it starts working, it works.

By the end of my first week, I felt like a new version of me was waking up. Lighter. Sharper. Clearer. And I haven't had a key lime pie since. Not even a craving.

Your body knows when you're lying to it. It also knows when you've finally decided to love it back.

TRINITY isn't just a product. It's a process. It's an invitation to live differently, eat intentionally, and honor the vessel that carries your purpose.

So as you begin your own journey, remember this:

I treat my body like royalty because it is the temple where power lives. I clear out what's expired. I nourish what's true. And I honor myself with every choice I make. This is not a trend. This is my transformation.

You're not just detoxing. You're making room for the best version of yourself.

~ T-Que Winning

Appendix

TRINITY USAGE DETAILS

DISCLAIMER

TRINITY is created to engage one in better health practices intended for maintenance of nutritional health.

At first this information may seem overwhelming. Get organized and follow all instructions day-by-day. An Easy-to-follow calendar is on the inside of every box top of TRINITY.

DAY 1:
GOOD GREENS Formula #1
Hawaiian Spirulina
Alkalinize. Energize. Nourish.

Instructions:

1. Take 10 Good Greens Tablets every day with food BEFORE 3PM.

2. Tablet may be chewed or dissolved for optimum absorption.

3. Drink 8-10 glasses of Alkaline, Lemon, or Cucumber water per day BEFORE 8PM. **GO TO BED BY 10PM EVERY DAY.**

4. Suitable for all ages and conditions.

- Ages 10-15 Maintenance dose for all ages because children should NOT detox.
- Ages 16+: Take 10 per day (Detox Dose)
- Ages 10-15: Take 5 per day (Maintenance Dose for all)
- Ages 5-9: Take 2 per day (Maintenance Dose)

DAY 2:
GOOD GREENS Formula #2
Chlorophyll
Balance. Detoxify. Purify.

Instructions:

1. Drop 1 capsule of Good Greens Formula #2 Chlorophyllin Capsule into a 500ml (16.9oz) bottle of water, dissolve and consume BEFORE 3PM.
2. Take 10 Good Greens Formula #1 Hawaiian Spirulina Tablets with food BEFORE 3PM.
3. Drink 8-10 glasses of Alkaline, Lemon, or Cucumber water per day BEFORE 8PM.
4. Suitable for all ages and conditions.

DAYS 3-7:
GOOD RIDDANCE
Parasite & Deworming Herbal Complex

Instructions:

1. Take 3 capsules of GOOD RIDDANCE upon waking on an empty stomach for 5 days.
2. Eat within 15 minutes of dosing.
3. Take GOOD GREENS Formulas #1 and #2 as directed.
4. On day 7, take the last GOOD RIDDANCE then **STOP**.
5. Not suitable if under age 18, pregnant, or breastfeeding.

-AND-

GOOD & CLEAN COLON
Herbal Colon Cleansing Complex

Instructions:

1. Take 2 GOOD & CLEAN COLON capsules preferably with Dinner with the last 2 full glasses of water for the day to keep colon pathway open for Parasites to escape and to have a smooth evacuation by morning.
2. Expect movement within 8-12 hours.*
3. ***Everyone varies, adjust time taken based on body response and schedule.***
4. Not suitable if under age 18, pregnant, or breastfeeding.

DAYS 8-12:

Instructions:

1. Take 10 GOOD GREENS Formula #1 Tablets every day with food BEFORE 8pm

2. Take 5 days off from, GOOD RIDDANCE, and GOOD & CLEAN COLON.

3. Drink 8-10 glasses of Alkaline, Lemon, or Cucumber water per day BEFORE 8PM.

DAYS 13-17:

Instructions:

1. Repeat all GOOD GREENS, GOOD RIDDANCE, and GOOD & CLEAN COLON steps from Days 3-7 to sweep out the remaining Parasites left behind or hiding in cracks and crevices.

2. On day 17 take the last GOOD RIDDANCE and GOOD & CLEAN COLON then **STOP**.

DAYS 18-21:

Instructions:

1. Take GOOD GREENS Formulas #1 and #2 as directed in Step 2.

2. Drink 8-10 glasses of Alkaline, Lemon, or Cucumber water per day BEFORE 8PM.

GET SET FOR SUCCESS
*GET ORGANIZED by placing a copy of the schedule on the fridge as a reminder of next steps.

TRINITY is designed to be most effective at official changes of seasons when Parasites are in the birthing cycle: 21 March, 21 June, 21 September, 21 December.

However, if a health issue is present or persistent, TRINITY can be taken any time and repeated at the next seasonal change to sweep out the Parasites born during the change of season.

*If your system is feeling overwhelmed by the Detoxification process, **STOP** the full doses for 2 days and resume at half of the dose.

*If weight is less than 100lbs (45.35kg) use half the dose.

*Drink half of body weight in ounces daily (i.e. 200lbs = 100oz of water) and only drink Alkaline, Lemon, or Cucumber water, Herbal Tea, Smoothies, or fresh juiced Juice.

*Exercise daily by taking a walk outdoors and breathing deeply.

*Bathe every night with a natural soap. Brush Teeth with a natural toothpaste at least 3x per day with focus on tongue, cheeks, crevices between teeth and gums.

SHOPPING LIST:
Fresh Vegetables and Fruit for eating, juicing, salads and smoothies (avoid Frozen vegetables and canned fruit during this process)

Organic Chicken, Wild-Caught Fish, Turkey, Dried Beans, Nuts, Raw Honey, Organic Maple Syrup, Stevia without Erythritol, Monk Fruit, Coconut Sugar

Snacks: Guacamole, Hummus, Organic Tortilla Chips, Nut Butters

Oils: Extra Virgin Olive Oil from the First Cold Press, Organic Coconut Oil, Avocado Oil, Real Butter

*NO-NOs:

Sugar (it feeds the Parasites you are eliminating!!)

Caffeine: Coffee, Black/White/Green Tea, Sodas (it deposits acid residue -vs- alkalinity)

Artificial Sweeteners (deposit acid crystals)

Beef, Pork, Ox Tails, Goat (all contain Uric Acid)

Cow Milk, White Pasta, White Bread, White Rice (all create a warm, sticky environment in the gut for Parasites to flourish)

White Products: White Bread, White Rice, White Pasta, White Flour, White Sugar

Oil: Vegetable Oil, Canola Oil, Margerine, Butter Spreads

During this detox, if you miss a day, get back on track. If you fall down with one of the NO-NOs...get back up!

CONGRATULATIONS on Step One of your Wellness Journey! Upon completion, your body will be well-nourished, hydrated, cleansed, and Parasite-free.

Grab an accountability partner to complete this program together. There is a war between desire and discipline. It takes discipline to reach for what we know is right in our weakness.

Email me your Health Praise Reports, I would love to hear from you: DrBrookshire@outlook.com.

I have hope that there is still a fight in us all to attain Perfect Health for the sake of our futures.

...And if I had to say Amen, I think I'd put one right there.

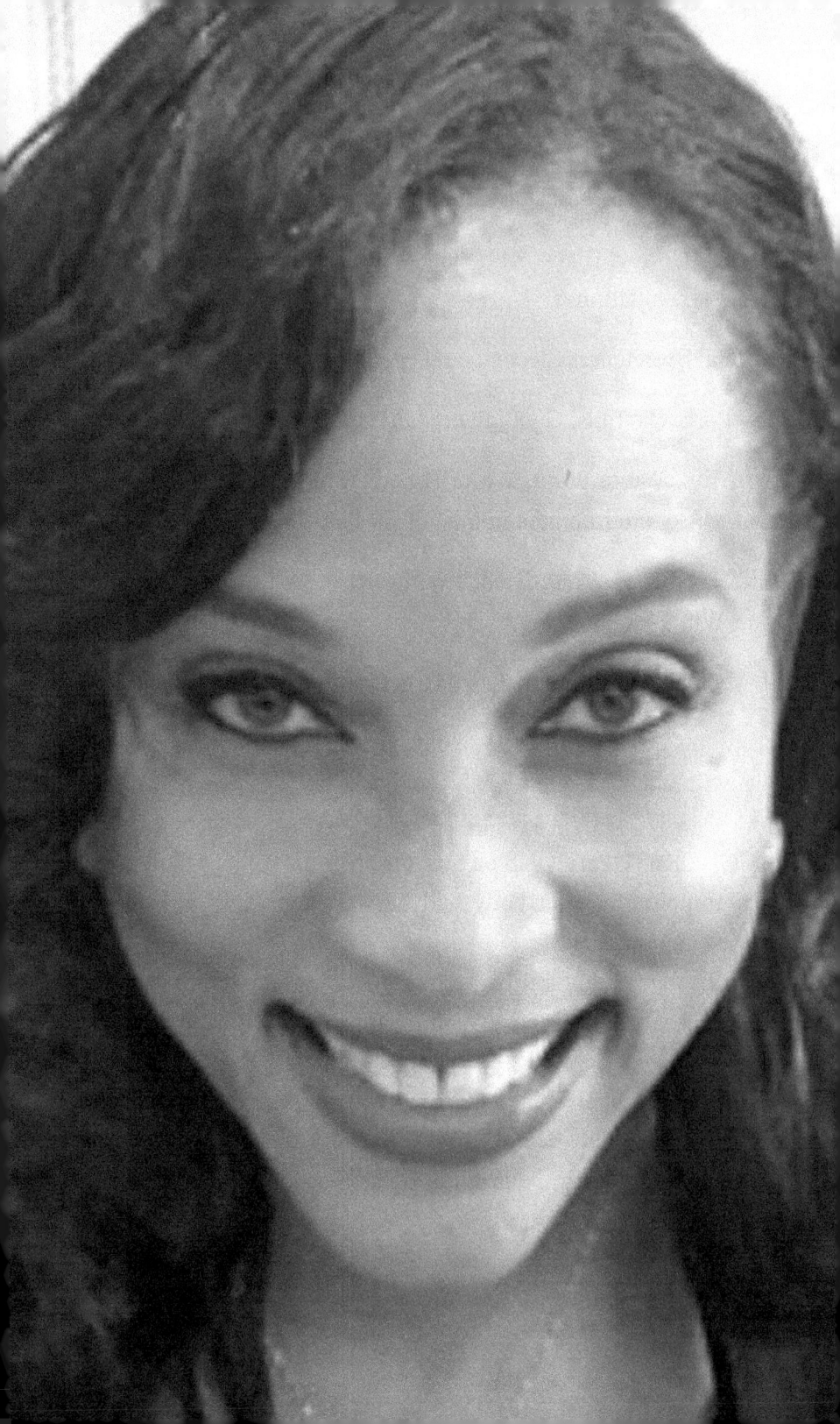

About the Author

Dr. LaJoyce Brookshire will quickly tell you she's God's Girl, a full-time wife and mother, licensed and ordained Pastor, Doctor of Naturopathy, Master Herbalist, New York Times Bestselling Author, Podcast Host of "ASK THE GOOD DOCTOR", College Professor, and Co-Creator of the TRINITY 21-Day Detoxification Program. Affectionately called "The Good Doctor", she treats many how to Attain, Maintain, and Reclaim ones Perfect Health using everything in nature. With ten concurrent bestselling books, today, Dr. Brookshire teaches corporations and groups worldwide about better health practices. Once a high-powered Entertainment Publicist during music's Golden Era to artists like The Queen of Soul Aretha Franklin, Usher, Toni Braxton, The Notorious B.I.G., Faith Evans, and Whitney Houston to name a few. LaJoyce is Co-Creator of the Women Behind The Mic: Curators of Pop Culture Book Series, Docu-Series, Lecture Series, and Curriculum featuring women who worked behind the scenes with the most iconic artists and brands of all time. Dr. Brookshire lives in Pennsylvania with childhood sweetheart husband Gus, also a Pastor, and together they have a daughter who is a professional Dancer and Choreographer.

Author Photo:
Elijah (Farmer) Muhammad
EM Photography

Scan here to
purchase TRINITY

www.ingramcontent.com/pod-product-compliance
Lightning Source LLC
Chambersburg PA
CBHW071247020426
42333CB00015B/1662